DRUGS AN
YOUR BRA

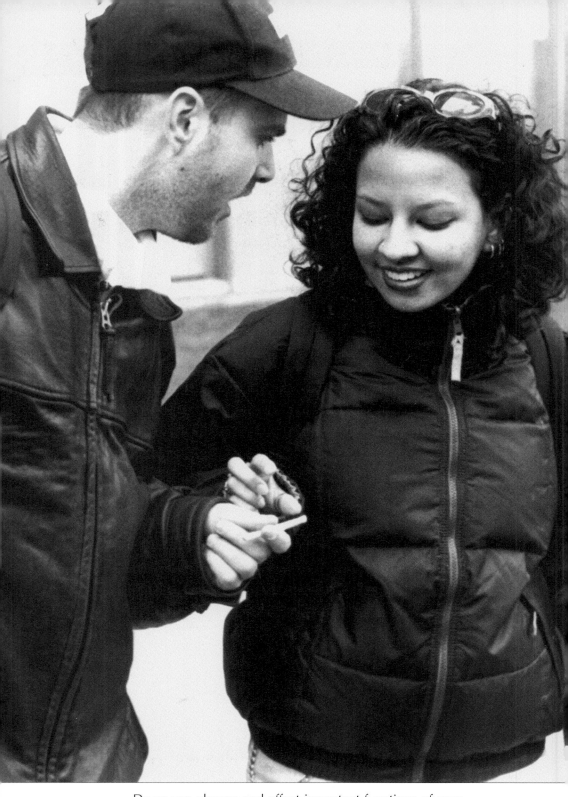

Drugs can change and affect important functions of your brain and your body.

HAZELDEN/ROSEN DRUG ABUSE PREVENTION LIBRARY

DRUGS AND YOUR BRAIN

Beatrice R. Grabish

A HAZELDEN / ROSEN Book

The people pictured in this book are only models. They in no way practice or endorse the activities illustrated. Captions serve only to explain the subjects of photographs and do not in any way imply a connection between the real-life models and the staged situations. News agency photos are exceptions.

The author would like to thank Ann Buczkowski and Lisa Williams-Hemby, Ph.D. at the Treatment Research Center, Department of Psychaitry at the University of Pennsylvania in Philadelphia.

Published in 1998 by the Rosen Publishing Group, Inc.
29 East 21st Street, New York, NY 10010

Copyright © 1998 by the Rosen Publishing Group, Inc.

First edition

This edition published in 1998 by Hazelden
PO Box 176, Center City, MN 55012-0176

Library of Congress Cataloging-in-Publication Data

Grabish, Beatrice.
  Drugs and your brain / Beatrice Grabish — 1st ed.
    p.   cm. — (The drug abuse prevention library)
  Includes bibliographical references and index.
  Summary: Discusses how the brain functions, the effects of drugs on
    the brain, how drug use can lead to addiciton, and where to get help.
  ISBN 1-56838-214-6
  1. Brain—Effects of drugs on—Juvenile literature. 2. Psychotropic
    drugs—Juvenile literature. 3. Drug abuse—Complications—Juvenile
    literature. [1. Brain—Effect of drugs on. 2. Drugs. 3. Drug abuse.]
  I. Title. II. Series.
  QP376.G685 1997
  616.86—dc21   97-26168
                                                               CIP
                                                               AC

Manufactured in the United States of America

Contents

Introduction

"If you take drugs you'll go crazy and shoot people!"
"Come on, just try it, drugs will make you feel good."

Many people have different attitudes toward drug use. Some people may try to convince you that drugs are terrible, while others will tell you that drugs are okay.

As a teenager, you are at the greatest risk for drug or alcohol abuse than at any other time in your life. It is estimated that 3 million teenagers are problem drinkers and 400,000 need treatment for drug abuse. This book will look at the process of abuse and addiction in the brain. It will also discuss the dangers of using drugs, and how to get help if you have a drug problem.

Drugs affect the central nervous system. It is this system that helps us gather and process information from the outside world. It is also responsible for our emotional and physical responses to our environment. This book will show you how drugs can alter the normal function of the brain and lead to physical and psychological addiction.

Scientists have made great advances in understanding brain function. As a result, a number of drugs have been developed to treat such conditions as depression and anxiety. While these prescription drugs can improve the patient's quality of life, the use of illegal drugs can have just the opposite effect. Repeated use of illegal drugs can actually alter the normal chemical balance in the brain. This can result in a physical dependence on the drug.

Drug abuse and addiction are serious problems. This book will focus on changes in brain function produced by drug use and abuse. A number of resources will also be provided for those who have a drug problem and need help.

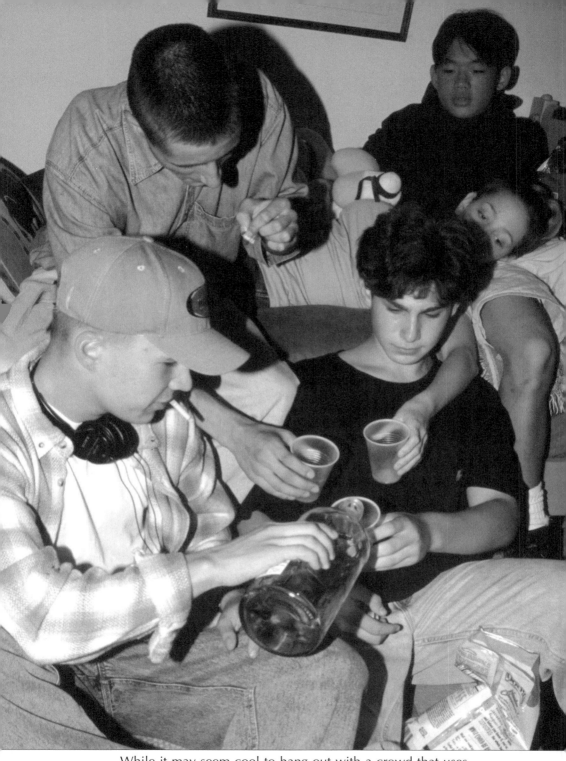

While it may seem cool to hang out with a crowd that uses drugs, you may be risking your health or your life.

CHAPTER 1

Tanya's Story

*T*anya was fourteen when she started using drugs. At her new high school, Tanya wanted to find a group of friends who would accept her.

The druggies seemed laid back and cool at first. They gave Tanya her first joint. Soon Tanya was one of the gang and was getting stoned with her new friends after school in the parking lot. On Fridays, she would cut classes and sneak out to be with her friends. They would sit in someone's car and pass around a joint. Everyone would take a couple of hits before they went back in to watch the basketball game in the gym. Tanya would sit on the bleachers and giggle as the players

10 | *dribbled the ball down the court. Her head felt like it was full of pins and needles.*

On the weekends, Tanya was invited to drinking parties. Her friends would gather in city parks or at the houses of friends whose parents were out of town. Because she already had the reputation of being a "stoner," Tanya was always invited to smoke pot at these parties.

One night, Tanya was really drunk and stoned. She stumbled around and slurred her words. Her eyes were glazed over and she often lost her balance.

The police came to break up the party. Everyone was jumping out of windows and running outside. Tanya couldn't run far and none of her friends waited around for her. Tanya was taken to the police station for questioning. She was issued a citation for dis-orderly behavior and underage drinking. The police suspected that she was on drugs as well. They called her parents and asked them to come to the station to pick up Tanya.

After that night, Tanya vowed that she would clean up her act. But she didn't realize just how hard that would be. When she re-turned to school, everything seemed to remind her of drugs. When she passed the parking lot at school, she wanted a drag off a joint. Even the bleachers in the gym triggered a craving to get high. Tanya doubted that she would be able to make it through the day without getting high.

Even though Tanya told herself that she wanted to stop, it was as if her brain were telling her the opposite. The longer she tried to stay away from drugs, the more she wanted them. Soon Tanya returned to her old group of friends and went back to smoking pot.

Tanya and her parents didn't realize that she needed professional help for her drug addiction. Quitting a drug habit also means changing your lifestyle. Tanya had adopted a certain lifestyle and a group of friends that accepted drug use. She needed to find a new group of friends and new activities to take the place of the drugs in her life.

To understand what was happening inside Tanya's brain when she got high, and to understand how she became addicted to drugs, we must first look at a healthy brain and how it works.

CHAPTER 2

The Healthy Brain

*H*umans have a central nervous system made up of the brain and spinal cord. The basic building block of the nervous system is the neuron, or nerve cell. The human brain has about one trillion neurons. Neurons communicate with the rest of the body by sending and receiving chemical messages. They collect information from the outside world and send the information to the brain to interpret. Neurons are also important in learning tasks and storing memories.

The human brain is made up of

numerous specialized areas that control

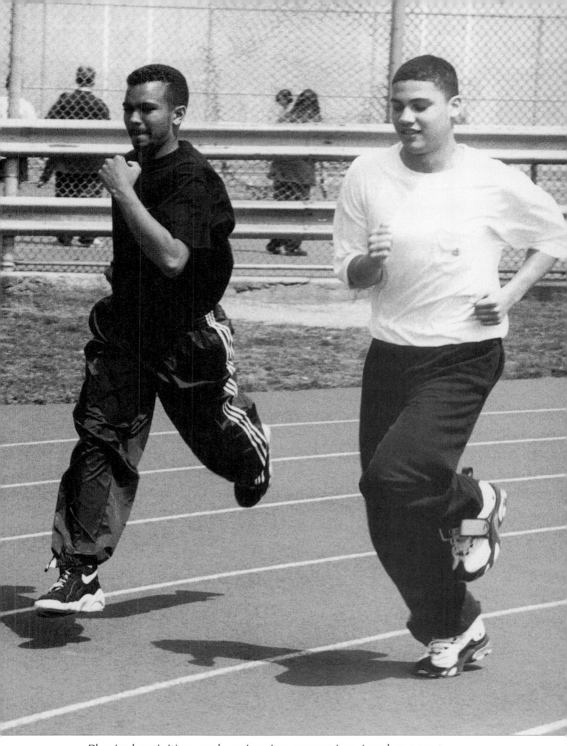

Physical activities, such as jogging or running, involve a part of the brain called the motor circuit, which is part of the frontal lobes.

14 | different functions. The brain is divided into a number of regions, each responsible for a particular activity or function.

The Basics

The portion of the brain closest to the spinal cord is called the brain stem. It controls basic functions such as heart rate, breathing, eating, and sleeping.

The Senses

Above the brain stem lies the cerebral cortex, which is responsible for thought, memory, and perception (how we see, hear, and feel things). The cerebral cortex is divided into two parts, or hemispheres. The right hemisphere largely controls a person's creative activities while the left hemisphere controls language and logical activities. There are dozens of specialized areas in the cortex that deal with specific functions. Most of the cortex is devoted to the five senses that allow humans to see, hear, taste, smell, and touch. The prefrontal lobes of the cerebral cortex (in both hemispheres) are the centers of reason, emotion, and judgment. The frontal lobes, which contain the motor cortex, are important in controlling movement.

Survival and Emotions

The limbic system is a set of brain structures that control our emotions and motivations. The limbic system connects our emotions to the cortex, which deals with the outside world. This connection allows us to experience feelings. These feelings are affected by our actions and by what we perceive in the outside world. Drugs act directly on the limbic system, which can alter our behavior.

Neurotransmitters: Chemical Messengers

Messages move through our brains from neuron to neuron. Neurons "talk" to each other by releasing chemicals called neurotransmitters. Each different kind of neurotransmitter is responsible for carrying a different signal. Some tell you when you feel pain; others tell you when you feel good. Each brain cell, or neuron, contains about fifteen neurotransmitters.

When you feel happy, your neurons release a neurotransmitter called dopamine. When you feel panicked, your neurons release a neurotransmitter called epinephrine, which triggers a "fight-or-flight" response. When you have a

16 | "runner's high," your brain is releasing neurotransmitters called endorphins, which make you feel good.

Neurotransmitters are released thousands of times a second. They deliver their messages and then return to the brain cells that originally sent them. Neurotransmitters can be used over and over again to carry other messages.

Every brain cell has a delicate balance of neurotransmitters, and each person has his or her own individual balance. This balance of neurotransmitters provides the chemical basis for his or her personality, talents, and ability to survive physical and psychological challenges.

Only when the brain has a correct chemical balance can it fully remember, concentrate, learn, coordinate, and cope.

Dopamine: The Main Neurotransmitter

Dopamine is an important neurotransmitter believed to regulate emotions and movement.

Dopamine is released when you ace a test, rest after a hard day, or win a basketball game. Mood-altering drugs that make you feel good increase the amount of dopamine in your brain. When dopamine can't be released, or when there is too

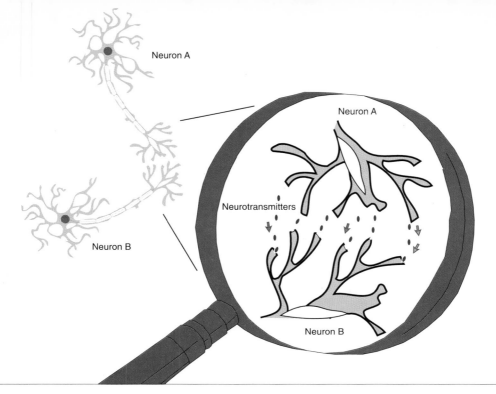

Neuron A

Neuron A

Neurotransmitters

Neuron B

Neuron B

Neurons communicate with each other by releasing chemical messengers called neurotransmitters. Neuron A releases its neurotransmitter which activates special receptors on neuron B (see inset). This process occurs millions of times per minute in the brain.

little dopamine in the brain cells, we feel depressed and unfulfilled.

The Dopamine Pleasure Circuit

The physical feeling of pleasure is one of the most basic human feelings. Humans learn to do those things that bring pleasure and avoid those things that cause pain. It is pleasure that makes us want to eat and drink, have sex (to have babies and increase the population), sleep, and seek shelter.

18 Pleasure, or what scientists call reward, is very powerful. If you do something that makes you feel good, your brain is chemically programmed so that you do it again and again. Mice and monkeys can easily learn to press a lever for food. Eating the food turns on their pleasure centers. Once the behavior is learned, the animal will repeat the action that produced the food. This entire process is an automatic brain function.

The brain has a specialized pathway of nerve cells to relay messages about pleasure. Dopamine plays a major role in this pleasure circuit.

Scientists have recently discovered that many drugs, such as marijuana, caffeine, alcohol, and cocaine all activate the dopamine pleasure circuit. This circuit also mediates the pleasurable feeling from food or sexual activity.

Drugs and the Pleasure Circuit

Certain substances, including many drugs, activate the brain's pleasure center, or circuit. Unfortunately, the more a person uses drugs to get that feeling of pleasure, the more he or she learns to repeat the drug-taking behavior, and the more the brain depends on drugs.

The main reason that people keep using |
drugs (even if they want to stop) is that drugs make them feel good by directly turning on the pleasure circuit. This is also one reason why drug addiction is so difficult to treat. Addicts find that only drugs can affect their pleasure circuit. In fact, animals trained to press a lever for food will abandon food and water for a drug.

Drug addiction is a disease that alters the way the pleasure center, as well as other parts of the brain, function. By directly turning on our pleasure circuits, drugs trick the brain into thinking that they are just as important as food and other necessities.

Jeremy's parents went out of town one weekend and his older brother Jason threw a big party at their house. Jeremy wasn't surprised that all the kids were drinking beer, but he was surprised that some of them were snorting cocaine. He had only seen cocaine in the movies.

"Hey, Jeremy," said Jason's girlfriend Cara. "Do you want to try this?" Jeremy walked over to where Cara and some of her friends were sitting. He heard them giggling and whispering about "getting Jason's little brother high." Jeremy was embarrassed. If he

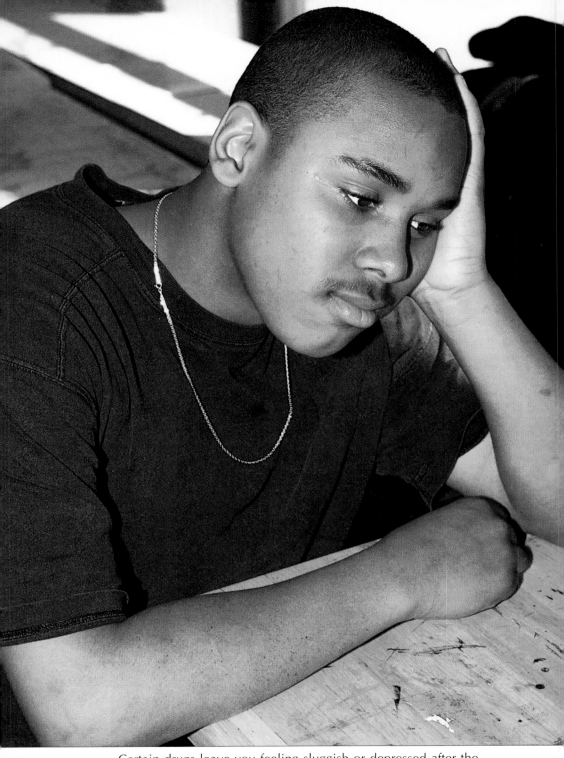

Certain drugs leave you feeling sluggish or depressed after the high wears off.

didn't try the cocaine, the girls would think he was a little kid. He sat down with Cara, and she showed him how to snort a line.

The cocaine made Jeremy feel like he had never felt before. He felt like he could do anything. He no longer felt like a gawky little brother; all of a sudden he could talk to anyone about anything. When he woke up the next day he felt like he had had the best time of his life.

The next week at school, Jeremy couldn't stop thinking about how good the coke had made him feel. He wanted that feeling again. He started sneaking into his brother's room to find his private stash. All he thought about in school was how he was going to get high later. The thought of getting that rush from cocaine was what got him through the day. Jeremy's parents finally found out about his drug habit when they caught him stealing money from their wallets.

Other Neurotransmitters

Serotonin is another important neurotransmitter which regulates our feelings and emotions. Serotonin is involved in sleeping, eating, and hunger, as well as agressive behavior. If serotonin levels are high, we feel relaxed. If serotonin levels are low or if the chemical is blocked in the brain cells,

22 | we may become aggressive or violent. Depression may also be a result of an alteration of serotonin levels in the brain.

Norepinephrine is the neurotransmitter most responsible for regulating the heart, breathing, body temperature, and blood pressure. Norepinephrine may also play a role in hallucinations and depression.

Acetylcholine governs muscle coordination, nerve cells, and memory.

Epinephrine turns on the "fight-or-flight" response when a person is in an emergency situation. This reaction prepares the body for strenuous activity. Epinephrine is also known as adrenaline.

Endorphins and enkephalins are two categories of chemicals. They help us handle pain, anxiety, and stress. Each category contains many chemicals, which are found in many places in the brain.

Other neurotransmitters control growth, allergies, the body's immune system, and personality traits.

The healthy brain contains a delicate balance of fifteen chemicals. In the next chapter, we explore how drugs affect that balance.

CHAPTER 3

The Brain on Drugs

*"Are you coming with us to smoke?"
Dave asked Christine at the party Friday
night. Christine was having a great time
dancing and talking with her friends. And
she already had a cool buzz going from a
couple of beers. But Christine followed Dave
and some other guys onto the fire escape.
Dave had a dime bag and a ceramic pipe.*

*Drunk and stoned, Christine wandered off
after the party without telling anyone that
she was leaving. She stood on the street with
her thumb out, trying to hitchhike back
home. Several cars passed before a police
officer stopped to pick her up. He drove her
home and talked with her parents.*

23

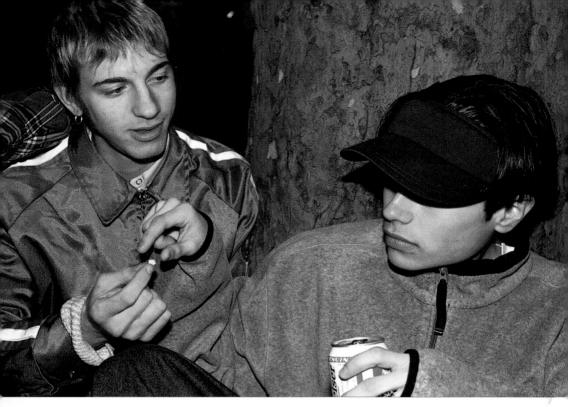

Drugs can affect your ability to make good decisions.

For a while, Christine was feeling really good. But her pleasure from drugs didn't last long. Normally, Christine would have had the good sense to get home safely. Marijuana and alcohol lessened her ability to make wise choices and take care of herself.

Most teens already know that drugs are chemical substances that can be habit-forming. Although it may seem cool to use drugs, it is important to know in advance how dangerous they can be. By looking at what happens in a person's brain when she uses drugs, it becomes clear how people like Christine lose control of their behavior, which can have dangerous, and even deadly, consequences.

Changing the Brain's Chemistry

One of the reasons that drugs can have such a powerful effect on the human brain is because they act directly on the brain stem and limbic system. These are essential parts of the brain because they control basic functions such as breathing, eating, and sleeping. These are also the functions that have helped humans survive as a species. Without the impulse to get enough sleep or reproduce through sex, humans would have died off long ago.

The human brain is much more complex than the brains of other animals. Humans have a cerebral cortex, which sends signals that help people think and judge right from wrong. When drugs act on the brain stem and limbic system, they can override the cerebral cortex. Drugs block off the part of the brain that helps us to make good decisions.

When a mood-altering drug enters the brain, the chemical balance of the brain cells is upset because the drug releases or blocks neurotransmitters. Each drug alters each neurotransmitter in specific ways, causing the changes we see in a

26 person's mood or behavior. Drugs also alter the chemical makeup of the brain and change the way it would normally respond to stimuli. This is why some people on drugs lose control of their coordination and behavior.

Some parts of the brain are more sensitive to drugs than others. For example, the cerebellum, which controls balance and movement coordination, is sensitive to alcohol. Valium mainly affects the midbrain, which controls emotional expression, hunger, aggression, and other functions. A barbiturate, on the other hand, will slow down the functioning of all parts of the brain.

Heather was known at her school for being a party girl. One night she and her friends Wendy and Liz crashed a fraternity party. In one room of the frat house, some people were playing a drinking game. Heather's friends urged her to join in, saying, "You'll totally win! Show these guys what you can do!"

An hour later, Heather found herself with a collection of empty beer cups at her feet. Her friends had disappeared. Heather stumbled out to look for them. She found a staircase and started to walk up. Wow, I'm really drunk, Heather thought, as she swayed and grabbed onto the banister. Some other people were coming down the stairs toward her, and she stepped out of the way. Heather misjudged where the step was, and lost her balance. Because the alcohol slowed down her reactions, she grabbed for the banister too late and fell. That was the last thing she remembered when she woke up in the hospital.

Different drugs affect the brain and the body in different ways. We will look at the most commonly abused drugs and their effects on the brain.

Narcotics and the Brain

Narcotics are drugs that cause sleep, lethargy, and relief from pain. Most narcotics are derived from opium and are called opiates. Opium comes from the seeds of the poppy plant. Opiates have been used throughout history to treat ailments ranging from common cramps and headaches to anxiety, epilepsy, strokes, and depression. Heroin, morphine, and codeine are all opiates. Opiates can cause physical dependency and a varying range of withdrawal symptoms.

Heroin, one of the most dangerous opiates, comes in a white to dark brown powder or tarlike substance, and can be

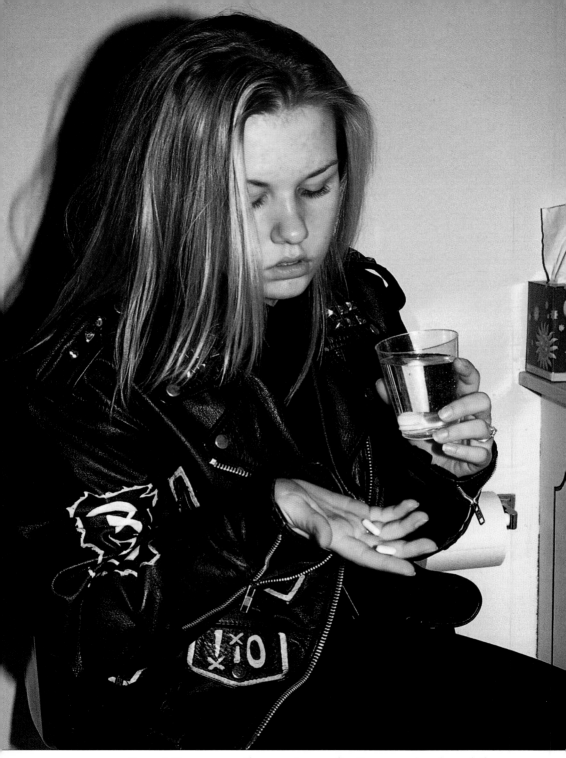

Prescription or over-the-counter medications can be abused if you take more than you're supposed to.

smoked, injected, or inhaled. Heroin is **29**
often referred to as horse, smack, or big
H. Heroin users call breathing in heroin
fumes "chasing the dragon." According to
a recent National Institute for Drugs and
Alcohol survey, 1 percent of high school
students have tried heroin. Heroin reaches
the brain in seven or eight seconds and
then latches onto special cells called receptors. Users, especially those who inject the
drug, experience a burst of euphoria, which
is often followed by drowsiness, nausea,
vomiting, watery eyes, and itchy skin.

Heroin use takes an enormous toll
on the body and is extremely addictive.
Short-term side effects include breathing
problems, nausea, vomiting, and consti-
pation. It is easy to overdose on heroin,
especially if it is mixed with alcohol. This
toxic blend can result in convulsions,
coma, and even death. Long-term users
who inject heroin develop skin abscesses
and vein damage. Those who become
dependent on heroin must take the drug
to feel normal. A break of only one day
can bring on withdrawal symptoms,
which include aches, chills, sweating,
muscle spasms, and weakness.

New studies show that heroin can
cause permanent brain damage. The New

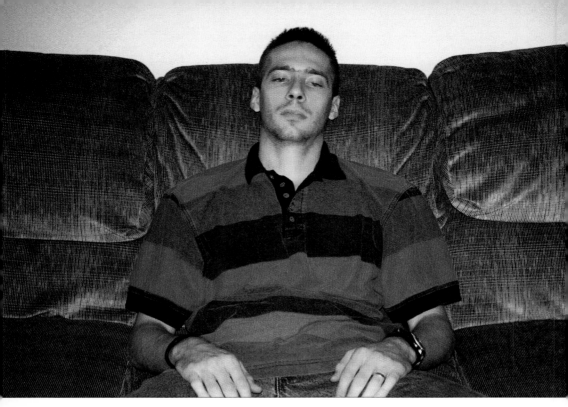

Withdrawal from a narcotic such as heroin could make you weak and very sick.

York State Office of Alcoholism and Substance Abuse found links between heroin smoking and an incurable neurological condition that can rob users of muscle coordination and speech. If untreated, this condition can lead to paralysis and death. Afflicted heroin users become clumsy, slur their speech, and wobble when they walk.

Depressants and the Brain

Depressants are drugs that slow down your body's reactions. They are often called "downers" because they slow down your heart rate, reflex time, and mental alertness. These drugs include alcohol, anti-anxiety and antipsychotic medications, sleeping pills, barbiturates, quaaludes, muscle relaxants, and sedatives. Most of these drugs are legally available by prescription and come in colored capsules and tablets. Street names for these drugs include goofballs, barbs, blue devils, yellow jackets, and ludes. According to a recent study released by the National Institute for Drugs and Alcohol, 6 percent of high school seniors report having used depressants.

Depressants can alter your brain's chemistry in a number of ways. Depressants slow down reaction time and can change your perception of reality. Mixing alcohol with other depressants can heighten their effects. Depressants can cause confusion, slurred speech, lack of coordination, tremors, and slowed heart and breathing rates. Large doses can cause respiratory failure, coma, and death. Taken repeatedly over a long period of time, depressants can become addictive.

Alcohol and the Brain

Alcohol is the depressant that is most accessible to teenagers. When drunk, a person may have trouble walking, slurred

32 speech, slowed reflexes, and bleary eyes. He or she may also experience behavior changes, memory loss, or an inability to concentrate.

In small amounts, alcohol acts similarly to a stimulant, causing some people to feel giddy or "up." But alcohol has many harmful effects on the brain. It can cause temporary memory loss and insomnia (inability to sleep). Alcohol also interferes with the brain's ability to produce REM (rapid eye movement) sleep. Adequate REM sleep is crucial to our physical and mental health. Also, some alcoholics suffer from a neurological disorder that can result in severe memory loss and hallucinations.

Even in small doses, alcohol can make you slur your words or stumble. It is also addictive. Alcoholism—the addiction to alcohol—has been shown to run in families.

Inhalants and the Brain

Inhalants are drugs that are sniffed to produce a high. They include household products such as glue, gasoline, and paint thinner; anesthetics such as nitrous oxide; and nitrites such as amyl nitrite and butyl nitrite. Abusers usually experience an immediate high followed by drowsiness, light-headedness, and other symptoms.

Inhalants depress the nervous system and have several serious effects on the brain. Long-term abuse can result in memory loss and difficulties with reading, writing, and math. After only one month of inhalant use, abusers can experience damage to the nervous system, including dementia (a deteriorating mental condition).

Stimulants and the Brain

Stimulants include cocaine, crack, amphetamines, diet pills, caffeine, nicotine, and antihistamines. All produce similar bodily reactions: your heart beats faster, your blood pressure rises, and your thoughts begin to race. Illegal stimulants are called speed because they cause all of your bodily reactions to speed up.

People high on stimulants have an artificial feeling of happiness that lasts anywhere from thirty seconds to two hours. Although users feel more alert at first, they soon become unfocused and jittery.

Many stimulants are highly addictive. They also produce a false sense of security among users. They trick you into thinking that you are focusing more than you actually are.

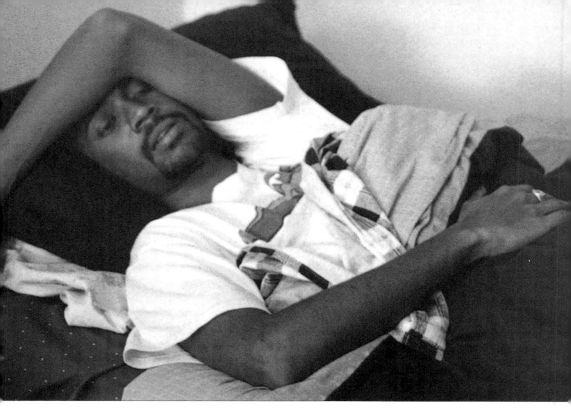

Depressants can affect your ability to sleep.

When a person uses stimulants, his or her brain becomes flooded with false messages. In time, the many false signals that stimulants send to your brain cells can cause serious damage to your body and can even result in death.

Cocaine and Crack

Cocaine is made from the dried leaves of the coca plant, and comes in a white crystalline powder form. Users can snort, inject, smoke, or swallow cocaine. It is most commonly called coke, but is also known as snow, nose candy, and rock. Cocaine enters the brain in seconds and produces feelings of euphoria, self-confidence, and power.

Recent statistics confirm that cocaine use is a growing problem among teens. Over 6 percent of high school seniors report having used cocaine at least once. Experts estimate that about 10 percent of casual users develop a serious habit.

Crack is a more potent form of cocaine that gets its name from the crackling sound it produces when heated. Crack can be bought in either white or tan pellets or as crystalline rocks.

Cocaine and crack increase one's heartbeat, breathing rate, blood pressure, and body temperature. A fast, intense high is often accompanied by feelings of excitement, sharpened concentration, and bursts of energy.

Cocaine is extremely addictive, even for first-time users. This means that the drug is in control. Cocaine's action on the heart and lungs can be very dangerous. It can cause an abnormal heart rate or even death in some otherwise healthy individuals. Even first-time users can die from just one hit of cocaine. Cocaine can also cause violent or erratic behavior and hallucinations. Long-term users often cannot stop sniffing even when not using

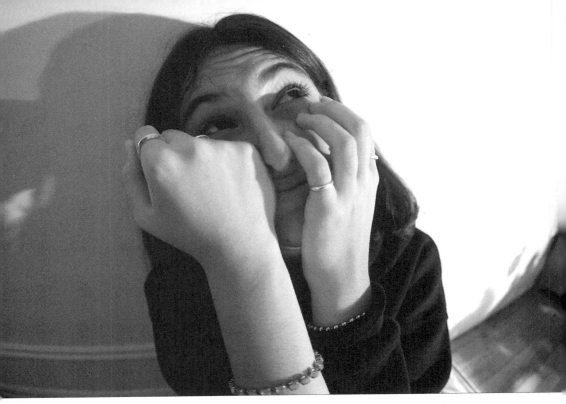

Hallucinogens distort your awareness of time and the things around you.

cocaine. This constant sniffing can cause ulcers to form in the nose lining or even cause the inside of the nasal structure to collapse. Cocaine users also develop abnormal tics in their tongues or eyes.

Cocaine withdrawal occurs after stopping the drug. Symptoms of cocaine withdrawal include sleep problems, irritability, depression, and anxiety.

Hallucinogens and the Brain

Drugs in this category include marijuana, LSD (lysergic acid diethylamide), mescaline, peyote, and PCP (phencyclidine). These drugs can alter a person's perception of reality. Tetrahydrocannabinol, or THC, is the main ingredient in marijuana. THC binds to the part of the brain called the basal ganglion where it can affect motor functions. THC is often used to reduce nausea and vomiting associated with chemotherapy, a treatment for cancer. Intense, continuous marijuana usage can cause memory defects.

These different types of drugs can stimulate the brain, depress the brain, or both. Some people try to get a mixed effect by first taking a stimulant and then taking a depressant to "take off the edge." This can seriously damage the brain, which experiences a roller-coaster effect from so many different signals. Repeated use of LSD has been known to cause changes in personality.

CHAPTER 4

Addiction and the Brain

Charlie headed toward his old neighborhood. It felt good to be free again. He hadn't used heroin since he had started his fourteen-month stint in the detention center. As the buildings of his old neighborhood came into view, Charlie broke out in a sweat. He gripped the wheel of his car as he tried to overcome a wave of nausea. But his feelings of panic became stronger as he realized that he was having the same withdrawal symptoms that he had experienced over a year ago in his detox program. Charlie thought he had kicked the habit for good, but now he felt awful. Charlie turned down a familiar alley. He knew how to get rid of this kind of sickness, and fast.

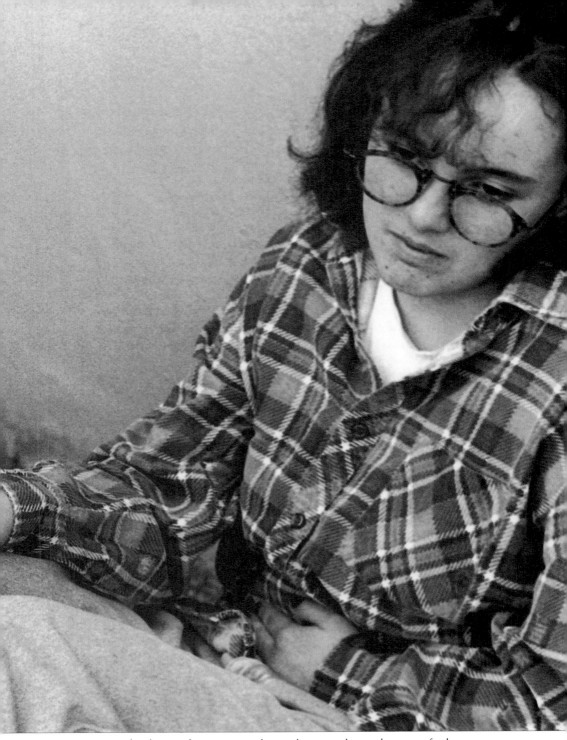

Your body can become so dependent on drugs that you feel sick if you don't use them regularly. Medical complications from drug withdrawal can even be deadly.

40   What was happening to Charlie? Can drug addiction be cured? Do clinical treatments and detox programs work?

Charlie, a recovered heroin addict, was having a relapse. He took drugs again to "cure" his sickness. Here we will discuss the causes of addiction and the reasons why it is so hard to overcome it.

Abuse vs. Addiction

Drug addiction and drug abuse are two different but related things. Drug abuse occurs when a drug is taken for a purpose for which it was not intended, or taken in a way or in an amount in which it was not meant to be taken. The U.S. government classifies drugs according to their potential for abuse and addiction. For example, heroin is not considered to have any acceptable use; therefore, whenever heroin is used, it is considered drug abuse. Even a drug like aspirin can be abused. If you take aspirin because you have a headache, you are using it for the purpose for which it is intended. However, if you take thirty aspirin for one headache, you are abusing it.

Drug abuse sometimes leads to addiction. Addiction occurs when someone loses control over the use of a drug and must use it frequently to feel normal. Addiction means that the addict is physically and psychologically dependent on the drug.

Before a drug addict actually feels the effects of the drug, the brain receives cues, or signals, that the drug is available. Drug users are "trained" to respond to certain cues in their environment which tell them that drugs are on the way. These cues can be either internal (inside) or external (outside). Feelings of anger or depression that often follow drug use are internal cues. External cues can include the smell of drugs or the act of rolling a joint. In Charlie's case, the sight of his old neighborhood triggered the craving for drugs. Besides the sight of the actual drug itself, other cues such as the people, sights, sounds, odors, and situations that are often involved with drug use tell the brain that drugs are available. An important part of any drug treatment program is teaching the addict how to cope with these drug triggers.

Recent studies have confirmed what scientists have suspected for a long time—that drug addiction is a disease based in your brain. Certain people have a specific genetic code that predisposes

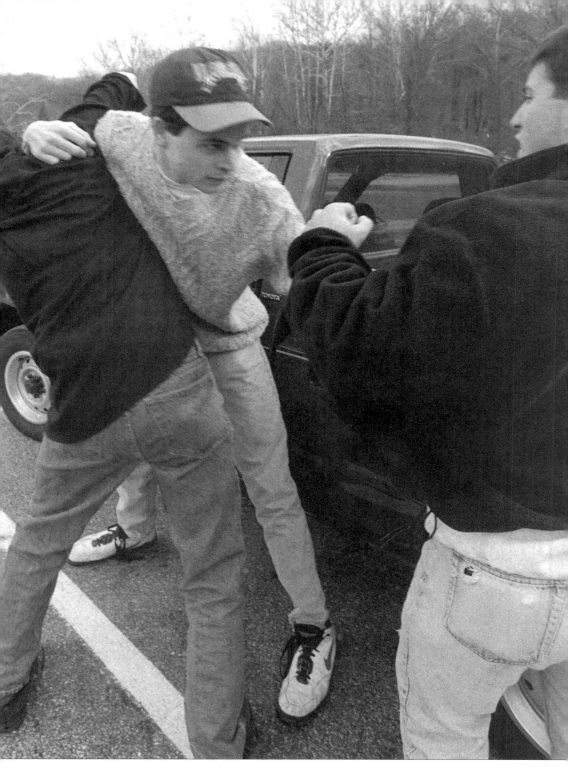

Drug use can often lead to violent or aggressive behavior.

them to addiction. Because of the nature of drug addiction, a quick "cure" is often not a realistic goal of drug treatment. The drug addict's lifestyle must also change, and this can be a lifelong process. People who are addicted to drugs have little control over their behavior. Drugs often take over the addict's life, and his or her only concern becomes figuring out when and how to get the next fix.

Physical Addiction

Once your body becomes used to a drug, it cannot function without that drug. Drug addicts do not feel normal until they have their fix. The constant presence of the drug has altered the chemistry of the addict's brain.

Like a thermostat, which controls the amount of heat in your house according to its temperature, the brain produces greater or fewer numbers of chemicals or neuro-transmitters to compensate for the extra chemicals from drugs that are in the brain. This is why so many drug users seem out of touch with reality, because drugs limit their ability to respond properly to the things that are happening around them.

Eventually the brain needs the chemicals found in the drug to reach the right

44 balance. Physical addiction happens when the brain depends on mood-altering drugs to function normally.

When the brain doesn't have the drug, it craves it. Craving is more than simply wanting or desiring the drug—your brain actually *needs* the drug. Scientists have recently been able to take pictures of the brain while it is experiencing a drug craving. This exciting development has allowed scientists to confirm that most addictive substances activate the same pleasure circuit in the brain.

After a while, your body also develops a tolerance to a particular drug. This means that with repeated use, the brain and body need higher and higher doses to create the same effect as the first few "hits."

Psychological Addiction

Psychological addiction occurs when a person becomes addicted to the way a drug makes him or her feel. An alcoholic might crave the way alcohol makes him forget his problems. A cocaine addict might crave the energy boost cocaine gives her.

Psychological addiction, unlike physical addiction, is often rooted in a person's insecurity. The addiction is a mental craving for the pleasure, or escape from pain, that the user gets from the drug. A teenager who has low self-esteem turns to drugs to feel better about herself. But the problems don't go away. Drug users develop a false faith that drugs can help them cope with a painful reality.

How Does Someone Get Addicted?

The brain maintains a certain level of neurotransmitters to keep a person feeling balanced. When a person takes drugs, the brain changes its chemical balance to compensate for the regular presence of drugs. For example, a cocaine addict's brain has an overabundance of dopamine. In response, the brain produces less dopamine. When a person stops using cocaine, withdrawal occurs. Withdrawal can cause intense feelings of sickness and pain.

Who Becomes Addicted?

Some people are more likely to become addicted to drugs than others. This has to do with the chemical balance in their brains.

Everybody has a unique chemical balance that affects the personality, good

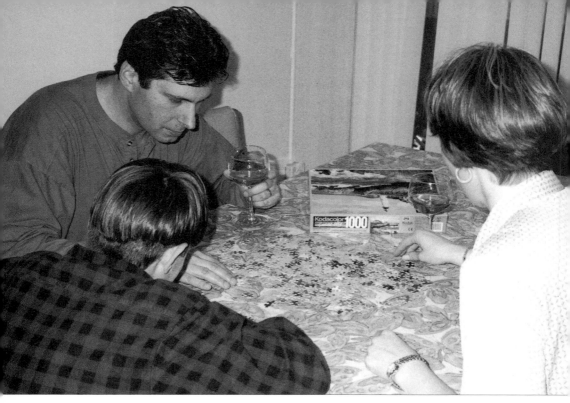

Your genetic makeup is similar to your parents' genetic makeups. This could affect your chances of becoming addicted.

and bad qualities, and ability to withstand physical and psychological difficulties. The combinations and patterns of a person's genes determine the right chemical balance for him or her.

Genes and a person's specific balance also affect the way a person's brain responds to the chemicals in drugs. Genes determine how fast a person's brain can reset its own chemical balance after drugs are taken. Just as your genetic makeup causes you to be short or tall, blond or brunette, blue-eyed or brown-eyed, your genetic makeup may also make you more likely to become addicted to drugs. For example, nearly 95 percent of cocaine users and 80 percent of alcoholics are children of chemically dependent (drug- or alcohol-addicted) parents. Even when children of chemically dependent parents are separated from their parents at birth, they develop addictions at the same high rate.

The Path to Addiction

Many teens who become addicted to drugs follow a similar pattern. By recognizing these steps, you can avoid falling into the drug trap.

1) **Experimenting.** Experimentation might start because of peer pressure, boredom, or curiosity.
2) **Forming a habit.** The person starts to use drugs again and again to feel good.
3) **Escaping from reality.** Drugs are often used to cope with stressful situations and painful or embarrassing feelings.
4) **Addiction.** Intense cravings cause a person to focus his entire life on getting the next fix. An addict may resort to stealing in order to get enough money for drugs.

48 | *Teen Drug Use: A Dangerous Trend*

Teens today have a dangerous attitude about drugs. They are more likely than teens in the past to accept drug use than to see it as harmful. They also report feeling more pressure to try drugs, according to a 1995 report issued by the Partnership for a Drug-Free America (PDFA).

More and more teens are taking drugs today. The National Household Survey on Drug Abuse shows that teenage drug abuse in the United States has almost doubled since 1992. This report also shows that overall drug use among those twelve to seventeen years old has risen almost 80 percent since 1992. The report attributed this increase in part to a new casual attitude toward drugs. This same survey showed that significantly fewer teens agreed with the statement "Taking drugs scares me." And the number of kids who said they didn't want to hang around with drug users fell 16 percent, from 55 percent to 39 percent. Disturbingly, more kids mentioned the "benefits" of drug use, like "Getting high feels good" or "Drugs help you relax and forget your troubles."

Reasons for the Growing Drug Problem

Why are more teens doing drugs? About 50 percent of teens surveyed say rock and rap stars make marijuana, heroin, and other drugs look cool. Drug use is often shown as no big deal—or as part of a glamorous lifestyle—on TV shows or in movies. There are fewer antidrug public service announcements on television than there were at the height of the "war on drugs" in the 1980s.

Teens are especially vulnerable to pro-drug messages, particularly if they have poor role models at home. When parents abuse drugs, they communicate the idea that drug abuse is okay. And it shows in the statistics. By fourth grade, 25 percent of children have tried alcohol. By high school, 55 percent have used alcohol or other drugs, and one-third get drunk once a week.

PDFA officials warn that as antidrug feelings decrease, drug use rises. For example, 67 percent of teens today believe that becoming addicted to marijuana is serious, compared to 75 percent two years ago. In addition, the number of teens who admitted to using marijuana in the past year jumped from 23 percent to 33 percent.

CHAPTER 5

Getting Help

*D*rug abuse and addiction are serious problems that affect not only the chemicals in your brain, but your friends and family as well. Fortunately, there are people who can help. If you or a friend or family member suffer from a drug problem, don't be ashamed to ask for help. See the help list in the back of this book for some options.

You have the power to prevent yourself from abusing drugs or developing an addiction. You can refuse to make drugs a part of your life.

Saying No to Peer Pressure
Although trying drugs can be tempting, it is important to stand up for yourself

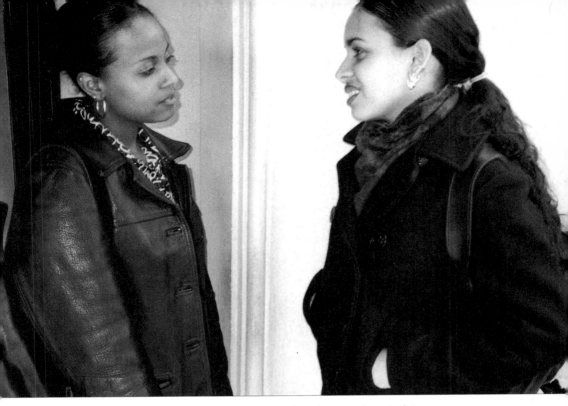

Friends can be very supportive as you break your drug habit.

and not give in to pressure to take them. Here are some things to remember when you feel pressured to take drugs.

- Be prepared. You must prepare yourself for situations where you might find yourself exposed to drugs. When you expect pressure at a party or with a certain crowd, you can come equipped with the answers you need to protect yourself. Or you may decide to avoid the situation entirely. It is up to you to decide whether or not you want to hang out with a drug-using crowd.

52

- Know the risks. When you have the facts about the dangers of drugs, it will be easier to resist the pressure and your own curiosity.
- Answer firmly. If you are wishy-washy about whether or not you want to use drugs, a pusher may take advantage of your indecisiveness.
- Have a full schedule. If you stay busy with extracurricular activities and events, you'll be less likely to find yourself in situations where teens are hanging out and using drugs.
- Use your head. Know who your real friends are. Anyone who pressures you to take drugs is not your friend, no matter how cool or inviting he may seem. Don't be fooled by smooth talkers.
- Respect yourself. Keep your goals in mind. Think about what's best for you and don't let anyone else lead you down the wrong track.

Helping a Friend or Family Member

Since they started high school, Steve and Rolando had gone to parties where kids were doing drugs. They both experimented at first. Rolando soon decided that drugs weren't for him. But Steve didn't stop. They still went to parties together, but Steve always ended up with the group of people who were doing drugs. Mostly he smoked pot. But a few times Rolando saw Steve snort cocaine. Another time he saw him smoking heroin.

Rolando tried to make a joke out of it. "Hey, you'd better quit that stuff before I have to drive you home in a body bag," he said after one party. Steve got angry. "I can handle it, okay?" he snapped. After that, Steve stopped calling Rolando. In the halls at school, he pretended that he didn't know him. Rolando was hurt, but he tried to blow it off.

Steve started looking worse every day. He was losing a lot of weight and he looked like he hadn't showered in days. One night, Steve's girlfriend, Maggie, called Rolando. She was crying. She said that Steve had punched her in a fight. "Was he high?" asked Rolando. Maggie sighed. "Are you kidding, Rolando?" she said. "Don't you know he's always high these days?"

Rolando knew he had to do something. The next day at school he talked to the school counselor and said he thought that Steve was addicted to drugs. She listened to him for a long time. Then she said that she was going to call Steve's parents. She told Rolando that he was helping to save his friend's life.

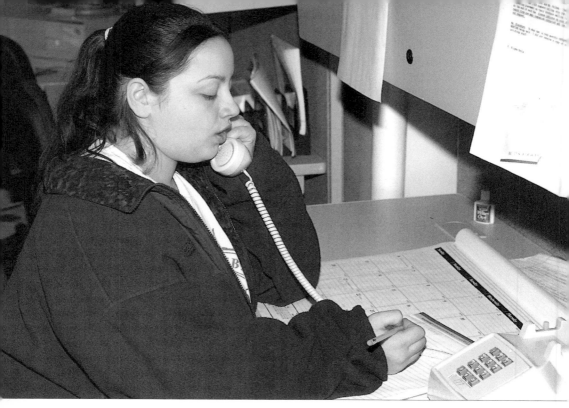
Help is available through drug hot lines or counseling centers in your area.

Rolando didn't see Steve at school the next week. Maggie told him that Steve's parents had checked him into a rehab program.

When Steve came back to school, Rolando avoided him. He was sure that Steve would be mad at him. But Steve cornered Rolando at his locker. To Rolando's surprise, Steve hugged him. "Thank you so much for what you did for me," Steve said. "I hope we can still be friends."

If you have a friend or family member who is in trouble with drugs, here are some ways that you can help.

- Confront her at a time when she is not high on drugs. Tell her that you think she may have a drug problem, and you want to help.

- Show that you care. Make it clear that you are concerned about her health and well-being. Do not pass judgment. Saying that you think she is stupid does not help. Also, do not unknowingly promote your friend or family member's drug problem by lying for her or giving her money.

- Anticipate denial. You have read about how drugs can alter a person's perception and ability to judge reality. Your friend or family member may refuse to admit that she is addicted to drugs. No one wants to believe that he or she has a serious problem.

- Seek professional help. It is not up to you to get your friend or relative to stop using drugs. Drug addiction is a serious condition that needs professional attention. You can get free advice by calling a toll-free drug hot line (see Where to Go for Help). Encourage your friend or relative to get reliable information and counseling through the organizations listed in this book.

56

- Talk to an adult you trust. This may be a parent, teacher, counselor, coach, or religious leader. Your friend or family member may be in real danger. If she cannot make rational decisions to help herself, an adult may need to step in to help.

Staying in Control

Pot, beer, cocaine, heroin, and other drugs fool the chemicals in your brain into behaving as if drugs are as important for your survival as food, shelter, or clothing. But you don't have to give drugs the opportunity to trick your brain. Staying clear of drugs will help your brain stay in control—and will help you stay in control of your life.

Drugs are powerful and can overrule your common sense. But understanding how your brain works and how drugs affect the brain can help you make an informed choice about your health and a future without drugs.

Glossary—
Explaining New Words

addiction The state of being psychologically or physically dependent on something.

cerebellum The part of the brain that controls muscle coordination.

cortex The most highly developed part of the brain. It controls emotions and judgment.

craving The physical or emotional desire for more and more drugs.

cues People, places, or things associated with drug use.

dopamine The neurotransmitter in the brain that is associated with pleasure.

drug abuse The use of a drug for a purpose for which it was not intended

58   or in a manner or amount in which it was not intended.

high   The feeling of enhanced pleasure one experiences after taking drugs.

limbic system   The part of the brain associated with the emotions and with motivation.

neuron   A brain cell.

neurotransmitter   Chemical messenger in the brain.

relapse   Falling back into patterns of drug use.

tolerance   The state a drug user reaches when he or she needs more and more drugs to feel the drug's effect.

withdrawal   The physical sickness a drug user undergoes when he or she abruptly stops using drugs.

Where to Go for Help

American Council for Drug Education
164 West 74th Street
New York, NY 10023
(212) 595-5810 ext. 7860
(800) 488-DRUGS

Center for Substance Abuse Prevention (CSAP)
Rockwall II Building, Room 800
5600 Fishers Lane
Rockville, MD 20897
(301) 443-0365

Cocaine Anonymous (CA)
3740 Overland Avenue, Suite G
Los Angeles, CA 90034
(800) 347-8998
Web site: http://www.ca.org/

60 | **"Just Say No" International**
2000 Franklin Street, Suite 400
Oakland, CA 94612
(800) 258-2766

Narcotics Anonymous (NA)
P.O. Box 9999
Van Nuys, CA 91409
(818) 773-9999

National Council on Alcohol and Drug Dependence (NCADD)
12 West 21st Street
New York, NY 10010
(800) 622-2255
e-mail: national@NCADD.org
Web site: http://www.ncadd.org/

National Drug Abuse Center
5530 Wisconsin Avenue NW
Washington, DC 20015
(800) 333–2294

National Institute on Drug Abuse (NIDA)
Public Information Department
5600 Fishers Lane, Room 10A39
Rockville, MD 20857
(800) 662-HELP
e-mail: information@www.nida.nih.gov
Web site: www.nida.nih.gov

Hot Lines

Center for Substance Abuse Prevention
Workplace Hot Line: (800) 843-4971
Cocaine Hot Line: (800) COCAINE
(262-2463)
National Federation of Parents for Drug-
Free Youth: (800) 554-KIDS
Youth Crisis Hot Line: (800) 448-4663

In Canada:

Alcohol and Drug Dependency
Information and Counseling Services
(ADDICS)
2471 1/2 Portage Avenue, No. 2
Winnipeg, MB R3J 0N6
(204) 942-4730

Alcoholics Anonymous
National Public Information Canada
P.O. Box 6433-Stn J
Ottawa, ON K2A 3Y6
(613) 722-1830

Council on Drug Abuse
698 Weston Road
Toronto, ON M6N 3R3
(416) 763-1491

For Further Reading

Berger, Gilda, and Melvin Berger. *Drug Abuse A-Z*. Springfield, NJ: Enslow Publishers, 1990.

Check, William A. *Drugs and Perception*. New York: Chelsea House, 1988.

Cheney, Glenn A. *Drugs, Teens, and Recovery: Real-Life Stories of Trying to Stay Clean*. Springfield, NJ: Enslow Publishers, 1993.

Drugs and the Brain. Bethesda, MD: National Institutes of Health, 1993.

Edelson, Edward. *Drugs and the Brain*. New York: Chelsea House, 1987.

Washburne, Carolyn K. *Drug Abuse*. San Diego, CA: Lucent Books, 1996.

Yoslow, Mark. *Drugs in the Body: Effects of Abuse*. New York: Franklin Watts, 1992.

Index

About the Author

Beatrice R. Grabish is a freelance writer and editor from New York. Ms. Grabish has studied at Georgetown University, Radcliffe College, and Columbia University. This is her second book for young adults.

Photo Credits

Cover 3-D illustrations by ©TechPool; cover still life photos by Michael Brandt; p. 30 by Carrie A. Grippo; p. 34 by Katie McClancy; p. 36 by Seth Dinnerman; pp. 39, 42 by Lauren Piperno; all other photos by Ira Fox.